ESSAYS ON EMOTIONS

TO HAVE AND NOT TO HOLD

AND

TO HAVE AND TO HOLD

Macklyn W. Hubbell

ISBN-13: 978-1530526987
ISBN-10: 1530526981

DEDICATION

This book is dedicated to the dearly beloved congregation of The Duncan Baptist Church.

ESSAYS ON EMOTIONS

Introduction   1

Emotions to Have and Not to Hold

1. Guilt   5

2. Anger   13

3. Fear   21

4. Grief   29

5. Anxiety   37

Emotion to Have and to Hold

Love   45

About the Author   53

ACKNOWLEDGMENTS

I am happy to express my appreciation for the loving support and contributions to this work by my wife, Bet. As I reflect on our upcoming 65th wedding anniversary, I can honestly say that the emotion I have most observed her demonstrate is love.

I would also like to thank my nephew, Steven Hubbell, who created the cover art (*Man in Mourning*) and provided editorial assistance for this book.

INTRODUCTION

Having been in the "marriage business" for decades, I have had countless numbers of couples to promise "to have and to hold from this day forward." I say "countless" because I have not kept a record of the marriage ceremonies I have performed; but the promises couples have made, with good intentions, I presume, was to remain in a state of a growing marriage "from this day forward." In other words, they were to have a growing, developing, meaningful relationship as long as they lived.

Fortunately for us as human beings, we have been created with a repertoire of emotions to exercise when it is appropriate and healthy. The range includes guilt, anger, fear, grief and

1

anxiety. When there is a valid reason for feeling responsible for a wrong doing or saying, guilt is appropriate. When there is a real present danger, fear is a normal emotion to feel or experience. When there is reason to have a strong feeling of displeasure, anger serves a purpose. When a loss of a loved one has occurred, grief is a healthy emotion or set of emotions to have; and when there is a painful uneasiness of mind, anxiety may be expected to rush through our emotional system giving us added energy to fight or flee.

Although these emotions may be healthy and expected, they are not to remain with us "to have and to hold" from the causative experiences forward unto the indefinite future. They are to be experienced as long as the emotion contributes to the recovery or wellbeing of the person.

The following essays will examine the experience of guilt, anger, fear, grief, and anxiety. What brings on these emotions? And how long should they remain dormant in our emotional system?

As a positive following to these emotions (those to have but not to hold) is the emotion of love. It is to have and to hold—never to be set aside, disregarded, or canceled. It is a foundational emotion in our system of feelings—always present even if weakened at times—and always present in us as the foundational emotion to be restored when weakened.

EMOTION TO HAVE AND NOT TO HOLD

NUMBER ONE: GUILT

1. GUILT

As human beings, we have a wide range of emotions like guilt, anger, and fear. For the most part, we express these emotions within appropriate boundaries; but there are those persons who hold onto these emotions well beyond the range of healthy appropriateness.

Let's take the emotions of guilt and examine its applied appropriateness. With the help of Webster, guilt is a feeling of responsibility for wrong doing. Obviously there are those persons who are diagnosed with an antisocial disorder and who have a pervasive disregard for the rights and personhoods of others. They do not care about the feelings of others; they run "roughshod" over anybody and everybody.

Most people, however, lie within the broad boundaries of emotional healthfulness. When they, therefore, violate others or society in general, guilt arises which is a normal response to a wrong doing. Take these examples: a person tells a deliberate lie about someone. There is little substance of truth in the lie, if any at all. It can be as simple as "Mary dates Harry and John when she is supposed to be committed to Albert." It is not only untrue but damaging to Mary, Harry, John, and Albert. The reality and circulation of such falsehood will or should produce a feeling of wrong doing on the part of the perpetrator. That is, guilt should be a nagging disturbing emotion.

In a marriage, a mate violates his/her commitment of fidelity. Arising in the violator should be a feeling of responsibility for a wrong act or acts. Or in a family, sibling rivalry gets out of hand and continues into adulthood. Damage will be done to the offended as well as the whole nuclear family. At some point or continuing over the years, guilt will or should make a violator feel an uneasy sense of responsibility.

Laws are made to protect us from others as well as society. These laws can be broken without the violator's being detected, charged, and punished. In such cases persons may carry guilt for having violated a law, possibly jeopardizing others of the society as a whole. Again, the emotion of guilt

The emotion of guilt should lead the person to recognize why he/she has such pervasive uneasy feelings. A healthy response to guilt is a recognition of "why I feel the way I do."

In addition to having guilt and recognizing why, the person should be led to take action. This may be in the form of a genuine admission of the wrong committed—word or deed. In no sense of the word should the apology be glib—an insincere expression of responsibility from the head—not the heart. It is easy to say "I'm sorry" without honest contrition.

I remember a traveler rudely breaking in a ticket line at an airport in Amsterdam. She said as she went ahead of us, "I'm sorry." Those of us who stood in line patiently awaiting our turn thought, "If you are indeed sorry, go to the rear of the line!

Prove that you are sorry."

In some instances of personal violations, as in the case of sexual inappropriateness (not when a child is born out of wedlock or venereal disease is contracted), the violator may do unnecessary harm to his current relationship by confessing. In lieu of confessing his/her earlier violation to his wife or to her husband, he/she should recognize that confession may lead to interpersonal disaster. If the violator is a person of faith, he/she should settle the issue with a forgiving God and move on without the deterrent of heavy, unhealthy guilt. Or take the case of a mother who admitted to her children, "I did not want you." The result of this guilt-led confession was permanent rejection felt by the children. The mother thought that her confession was necessary for honest healing; but in reality, it did permanent damage to the unwanted children—added, unnecessary emotional pain. Obviously it would have been better for all concerned if the mother had admitted their being unwanted to her priest or confessor—not the children.

As indicated above, guilt is a normal, healthy emotion which should be recognized or admitted to and followed with compensatory words or actions. On the other hand, guilt should not be brushed aside or buried in the subconscious. In either case, guilt, unresolved, will do emotional damage to the person—even though it was either pushed aside or buried.

Being a person of faith, I recommend strongly that guilt be dealt with in the context of one's relationship to God. After all, when matters are not resolved with others, one's relationship with God is interfered with: "if you do not forgive men their sins, your Father will not forgive your sins."

The bottom line is quite simple: Guilt is one of those emotions to have, but not to hold on to. Release it through appropriate action or deed; and then move on toward emotional healing.

EMOTION TO HAVE AND NOT TO HOLD

NUMBER TWO: ANGER

2. ANGER

Anger is an emotion which has a place in our emotional repertoire. A broad definition of this emotion is "a strong feeling of displeasure and belligerence aroused by a real or supposed wrong." I have discovered a couple of my expressions of anger. One was in grade school involving a classmate named Pat. We were on the playground during recess playing a quick game of soccer. For some reason, I thought Pat was violating my space. Instead of sorting out my feelings, I responded in anger. Immediately my anger caused me to double my fists. Neither his life nor mine was in danger. It was just low level anger. Fists flew and Pat landed on the ground. As I recall this incident of anger, it was more of a test of muscular strength. It lasted only minutes; and it was all over.

A decade or so later when I was a college sophomore, our house mother accused me of doing something I did not do—hollering out an "obscenity" from the bathroom. The house in which we lived across from the university library had a long hall from the front to the rear door. The bathroom was at the end of the "dog trot." Every time my roommate Jimmy exited the guy's restroom, he yelled, "Momma, come get me, I'm through!" The guys in the house thought it was hilarious; but the house mother did not.

In a round-about way, the house mother reported to Jimmy's uncle who reported to my family that I was the one who was shouting these words multiple times. I was reprimanded in "holy" language for speaking "un-holiness"—even though I denied vigorously having said it.

This made me angry with Jimmy's uncle for reporting to my family that I was the one yelling vulgar words. I determined that I would confront Jimmy's uncle when the opportunity allowed. It was a number of years before I finally had the chance to confront him. I was attending a professional conference along with hundreds of others. After a morning session, as I was leaving the conference hall, I noticed Jimmy's uncle sitting in a chair in a slouched posture. "Now is my chance!" I said to myself. As I approached him within ten steps, I realized that he was an old, sick man who had suffered a stroke. I stopped, turned, and walked away.

My anger evaporated immediately; but I thought how foolish I had been to harbor such anger; and furthermore how damaging my pent-up anger had been to me—not to Jimmy's uncle. Even though my anger may have been unwarranted, I neither expressed it in a controlled manner nor at an appropriate time.

At times—particularly closer to the event—I may have experienced teeth-grinding, clenching of fists, tightening of muscles, and even temperature changes—characteristic of pent-up anger. If I had thought about the offence on a daily basis, my anger would have produced hormones to temper the effects of my adrenalin flow; and it could have weakened my heart because of a stiffening effect on my arteries. Moreover, unresolved and locked-in anger could have led to potential liver and kidney changes as well as an increase in cholesterol causing anxiety, and even depression. According to a study of 13,000 subjects with higher levels of anger, coronary artery diseases can develop causing three times the risk of heart attacks. And some researchers speculate that chronic anger may even be more dangerous to one's health than smoking or obesity.

It may sound as if anger is a negative in our emotional repertoire. Yet, we are created by God with the potential of anger for reasons; and the basic reason is that anger raises our level of displeasure and belligerence aroused by a real or supposed wrong. As a person of faith, I am reminded that the Galilean's anger was exercised to drive money changers from the Temple. And it goes without saying that the Old Testament writers attributed to God a quality of anger or wrath.

Having the potential of anger, it behooves us to have a healthy personal understanding of anger and to exercise the expression within healthy limits.

Therefore, personal rules for healthy expressions of anger should always be in place:

1. Do not allow anger to be excessive and prolonged.
2. Delay personal action when one has a strong level of displeasure and belligerence aroused by a real or supposed wrong.
3. A delay in action when angry may lower the potential of extreme reaction even if it is as simple as counting to ten before acting.
4. Rule out being physical when angry, resorting to verbalization or healthy communication.
5. Bring anger to an end; do not allow oneself to carry it into the indefinite future.

The bottom line is as stated earlier: Anger is an emotion which we all have the potential for; but it is an emotion to have but not to hold on to.

EMOTION TO HAVE AND NOT TO HOLD

NUMBER THREE: FEAR

3. FEAR

Those of us who lie within the boundaries of normalcy will experience the emotion of fear, stimulated by one event or source. A few years ago Bet and I were sitting comfortably in our seats and with our seat belts buckled around us. The captain of our flight circled the Tokyo airport preparing, we presumed, for a normal, uneventful landing. Suddenly, a flight attendant, in a calm, confident voice said, "Make certain your seat belts are fastened and lean forward with your heads against the seat in front of you." Knowing something was wrong, but not knowing what, I lifted my head for a peep outside. On the runway below us I saw fire trucks, ambulances, and emergency personnel. In a matter of seconds, the aircraft hit the runway stopping on a virtual dime. After our abrupt landing, the captain said, "I apologize for the landing; the landing gear did not function, but the backup system did. Welcome to Tokyo."

Fear became the dominant emotion. Do we scream for help? Do we unbuckle and fall into the aisle? Or do we not let fear overwhelm us, remaining mentally alert and emotionally under control? We chose to do the latter.

On another occasion, we landed in Florence, Italy, in the early afternoon. I left Bet with Margaret and Pete Walker to head for the rental car agency while they proceeded to the carousel to claim our luggage. All went as planned—rental car running and baggage in our grips. We headed for the round-about just outside the airport. Instead of circling and going south, I circled and headed north. No big deal, I thought; I will exit and return to the freeway to head south. We passed through well-lighted tunnels one after another. We approached another tunnel where the lights did not function; it was like a pitch-black cave.

Since it was early afternoon, I had not located the light switch to turn on the head lights. I did have enough composure to stop the car, putting it in park position. No lights were ahead or behind us. In a matter of seconds, I located the switch and turned the lights on and moved ahead toward our destination. Of course, the dominant emotion was fear. Let it control us? Or keep our fear checked and controlled. We chose the latter and proceeded ahead—safe and sound.

Our son, Floyd and I went on safari in Kenya, sleeping and eating in tents. One early morning we decided to cross over a stream to check out the other side. As we walked cautiously, we were half way across the bridge when suddenly a family of baboons was on the opposite side of the bridge positioning to attack us. Their doglike muzzles were open, displaying their threatening fangs. Again, the potential emotion could have been fear. Instead, our muscles were energized and we backed away rapidly from the angry pack of baboons.

In the 1960s dramatic racial changes were in the making. As pastor of First Baptist Church, I privately and publicly called for our congregation to recognize that "all people are created equal by God and deserve to be related to as equals." It was a relatively mild position, but a positive one.

Naturally word of my position spread throughout Cleveland, which stimulated a minority of persons to have uncontrollable anger. Shortly after making my position known (equality and fairness), I entered the church on Monday expecting a routine day. I noticed the church mail on the credenza. As I sorted the pile of mail, I realized that one letter addressed to me had no stamp on it. Curiously, I opened it. Enclosed were a number of Life Magazine photographs with dead and wounded bodies strewn on the streets of a northeastern city. Scrawled in handwriting was an angry note which read: "Leave Cleveland or this will happen to you."

Fear was a potential feeling which the threatening letter could have aroused. However, in lieu of the emotion of fear, it was anger. Since it had been delivered by the postal authorities without a stamp, I reported the reception of the letter to federal authorities. It was discovered that a frightened (over racial disturbances) female in the general neighborhood had sent the letter. Case closed—no fear and my anger was checked. Notwithstanding, fear was a potential feeling the letter could have aroused.

In summary, fear is another of those emotions which normal people have the potential of personally experiencing. By the same token, it is an optional emotion. The emotion of fear serves us as an internal, emotional alarm system. When an experience or a situation causes apprehension or fear, he/she has several options: one is to be so overwhelmed to the extent that one's mind disconnects and fear takes over. Another option is to react to the experience with a spontaneous response like wild vocalization or irresponsible anger. Still, a better response to a fearful experience is to react in a nondestructive way. In other words, one's cognitive resources can kick in to determine the logical response.

For some persons, fear of anything and everything is a lifestyle. Any experience with which they are not familiar will create uncontrollable fear. To move from this mindset, persons must practice using their minds to determine a reasonable response. For instance, if seeing a snake creates fear, the mind should "kick in:" "This is not a venomous rattlesnake—only a harmless grass snake."

Now back to the premise: fear is a normal emotion or response to have under threatening situations, but not an emotion to "have and to hold."

EMOTION TO HAVE AND NOT TO HOLD

NUMBER FOUR: GRIEF

4. GRIEF

In the late 1960s, medical doctor Elizabeth Kubler-Ross penned a classic work entitled <u>On Death and Dying.</u> On the cover of the book appear these words, "What the dying have to teach doctors, nurses, clergy, and their families." After discussing the fear of death, she moves in the written direction of attitudes toward death and dying.

At the heart of her study, she describes the stages the dying go through: "...we have learned from our dying patients in terms of coping mechanisms at the time of a terminal illness."

The stages patients go through, according to her research, do not flow in smooth succession, but she discovered that patients move, at their pace, though these stages: *Denial and Isolation, Anger, Bargaining, Depression, and Acceptance.*

I have introduced this classic for a reason; and the reason is grief, whether related to the dying patient or those left "temporarily" on the other side of Jordon. Grief is a process which should result in acceptance. I have inserted the word "process" in the previous sentence because it is just that. It is a process which should have an ending—not a grinding, gnawing feeling that goes on *ad infinitum.*

It may be an unnecessary reminder; but I will take responsibility for redundancy. Grief occurs, obviously, when a two-year old dies from choking on a piece of beef. When this happens the relationship with one's family is severed—never to be had again. The reason of death may cause one parent to feel responsible: "Why did I not do more?" Or, "What could I have done differently?"

If a person has lived her three-score and ten and more and dies, someone outside the family may say, "She lived a full life;" nonetheless, the family of the deceased will go through a period of grief.

Death is not the only reason for grief; a loss of one's meaningful property may cause grief. For an example, a family business or home with lifelong personal treasures like pictures, antique furniture, or a wedding dress may go up in flames. Grief, no matter how short-lived, may set in.

Grief with a heavy dose of depression may occur when a person loses his job at age fifty-two. The prospects of another such job with equal or more pay may not be on the occupational or professional horizon.

No matter what the source of grief, the inception and process will move from shock and disbelief to anger, bargaining, and even depression. The duration of these stages will vary from person to person. For some a short period; and for others, a longer duration.

The final goal of grief is the morning light of recovery. Consider one of the above examples of grief, the accidental death of a two-year old. Even within the family, recovery will vary: siblings may take less time while the parents' length of recovery may take more time. Notwithstanding, time for healthy recovery will or should bring about stable recovery.

Recovery time under ordinary circumstances will move through the calendar year. Again, in the case of a death, birthdays, anniversaries, and holidays will come and go. As grieving persons move through these events, the intensity will or should be reduced.

Saying that grief with the passage of time will bring healthy recovery does not suggest that the person who has died will be forgotten. Another phenomenon called memory will be activated with greater meaning. After all, events and happenings come and go lasting only for brief times— an hour, a day, or a week. Healthy memories will help those who are moving into recovery to recall, reminisce, and enjoy the past relationships.

If painful grief is extended longer than a year or so, it will have gone beyond its healthy length of time. Becoming locked into grief beyond its intended time for healthy recovery causes serious internal as well as interpersonal pain. The pain one feels inside herself/himself can affect diet, sleep, and emotional stability as well as internal emotional pain. Interpersonal emotional problems can also develop.

For instance, in the case of a child's death, the mother's relationship with her other children can be seriously damaged; the husband or wife who does not pass through the healthy stages of grief may suffer from a breakdown in their marital relationship—incessant crying or unfair blaming creating distance or even separation or divorce.

The bottom line is that grief is designed by our Creator for us to move progressively from one stage of grief to another in the direction of recovery. Again, I want to emphasize that the person of death or whatever the source of grief is will not fade into oblivion, that is, the source of grief will not be forgotten or the loss will not be wiped from memory. The pain will be wiped away; but the pleasant memories will remain for recall.

Grief is an emotion to have but not to hold on to.

EMOTION TO HAVE AND NOT TO HOLD

NUMBER FIVE: ANXIETY

5. ANXIETY

From a psychiatric point of view (Diagnostic and Statistical Manual of Disorders), anxiety is a disorder which can be classified variously according to the presenting symptoms. These are some of the categories of anxiety disorders:

agoraphobia   *generalized anxiety*

Panic attack   *Post traumatic stress*

obsessive compulsive   *social phobia*

Moving outside the DSM, anxiety is a fear, disquiet, or worry over the known or the unknown. It is a complex emotion which we all have the potential of experiencing. Whenever there is a threat or perceived threat of danger, the human body can secrete hormones which will affect the whole body, physical as well as mental.

I had not experienced anxiety—that I recall—fear, yes, until I was working on my master of arts degree at the University of Houston. I was traveling back and forth from Houston to the small town of Wallis, our residence at the time. Examination and course requirements were overwhelming, I thought. My thoughts were incessantly focused on my academic goal. At times, I experienced shortness of breath and abdominal tightness; and my thoughts were on academic deadlines.

Not having had such feelings before, I simply labeled it as stress. As I reflect on it, I recognize that it was anxiety due to academic pressure. When I met assignments and passed all my scheduled exams, my anxiety was checked and brought under control.

A few decades ago, I boarded a Delta Airlines plane—one of my first flights. I was seated next to a window at night and saw what appeared to be fire in one of the engines. It was not; but at the moment I did not know that it was normal heat generated by the engine. For an hour or so I became anxious, fearing a crash.

Since my profession calls for public speaking and I can recall earlier in my career that when I was not adequately prepared, or thought that I was not, anxiety with its obvious symptoms appeared—shallow breathing, abdominal muscular tightness, and dryness of mouth.

The above experiences relate to an earlier period in my life when I did not know how to identify my unpleasant feelings. Later with acquired knowledge and awareness, I learned what to call my unpleasant feelings—anxiety. And, I might add, how to keep it under control.

Now back to the definition of anxiety: It is distress or uneasiness caused by perceived danger or misfortune. When anxiety is not overwhelming or disabling, it can rev one up or energize one for the assigned task.

But when anxiety is excessive, it can be debilitating. Reaching this level, it can become an anxiety disorder resulting in a panic attack causing a person to irrationally flee from the perceived

41

danger. Or in time can become lingering or generalized anxiety. When anxiety reaches this level of intensity, it is classified by professionals as a disorder requiring medication (perhaps) or verbal therapy.

The common variety of anxiety can be brought under control preventing it from rising to the level of a disorder requiring professional help or assistance. Recognized success at controlling anxiety can come from relaxation—the antithesis of anxiety. When a person feels the onset of anxiety, he or she should get in a relaxed, reclining position. In so doing, the person can exercise mind control, that is, encouraging one's mind to think of a tranquil scene in a park or the flow of a gentle waterfall, etc.

If one is not able to recline, deep breathing will help to bring relaxation—inhale to the count of 5, hold to the count of 5, and release to the count of 8 through the mouth. This will help to stabilize shortness of breath and balance the body's need for oxygen.

Since music (classical or any genre of soothing music) is so available, listening to comforting music will help to lower anxiety by mentally focusing on the music. Or for some, a relaxing diversion like drawing or painting will help to bring anxiety under control.

Exercise, walking particularly, will help a person whose anxiety level rises. If walking out-of-doors is not advisable, walking from one side of a one's residence to another brings relief. Or walking in a safe building like Walmart will help to reduce anxiety. Simply take an empty basket and stroll from one aisle to another. Pick up a loaf of bread for the basket if an empty basket calls attention to your stroll.

Anxiety is a potential emotion that all persons have. To repeat, it is a response to distress or uneasiness. And as long as it remains on a lower level, it is controllable. If it rises to the level of a disorder (however diagnosed), request for professional assistance is appropriate.

And, I might add, anxiety or the potential for it was not introduced to humanity in the twenty-first century. After all, Jesus counseled in the Sermon on the Mount not to worry about life in general—specifically food, drink, clothes, or even tomorrow. He was not condemning the anxious person; rather he was recognizing its potential and encouraging faith for life's essentials.

And so, anxiety or the potential for anxiety lies in us all. It serves as an alert signal when a real or imagined danger appears. Taking action in the face of the "red flag" is the preferred and healthy response as opposed to exacerbating the emotion.

EMOTION TO HAVE AND TO HOLD

LOVE

LOVE

In previous essays, I have written about emotions which we have or have the potential for, but not to "hold on to." There is still another emotion which stands apart from guilt, fear, grief, anger, and anxiety. It is an emotion, but it is one which we should hold on to – love.

The emotion of love is difficult to define because we use it in a variety of contexts: "I love lemon pie," "I love my mother," "I love spring weather," "I love dogs," and "I love my wife." Even Webster does not help us with its definitions-one and two: "a profoundly tender passionate affection for a person of the opposite sex" and "a feeling of warm personal attachment or deep affection, or its gratification."

In the context of this essay, love is the feeling one has for God and persons: "Love the Lord your God with all your heart…soul…and…, mind" and "love your neighbor as yourself." A refined definition of love from this point of view comes from the actual Greek word, "agape."

The word "agape" is a first century Greek word for love which has deep meaning. In the first place, it is committed love without any condition. I love you, not I love you "IF." There is no "IF" in agape. Once the love is given or freely offered, it becomes a permanent commitment. Once this love is given to another, it does not expect love in return: "I love you but I expect love in return." Even if the receiver of this love at some point in time rejects his or her love, this rejection does not nullify or cancel this love one has for another. Once this love is genuinely given, there is nothing the recipient of love can do to erase "agape."

The depth of this love sounds like it is humanly impossible to have and to give to another. According to my faith-understanding of God, when we have an agape relationship with God, He empowers us to love with this profound quality of love. In other words, we cannot love another or others or even God unless He endows us with the capacity to love with "agape-depth."

To repeat for emphasis, to have the agape quality of love, persons must have a transforming relationship with God who in turn endows us to have the capacity to love with this quality. Consider these relationships: The husband/wife and the wife/husband relationship may start with a potential for agape. In time this quality of love grows and develops. No matter what level this love is in the early "I do" stage, it always has the genuine ingredient of "I love you, no matter what!" This "what" may consist of "founded or unfounded anger" she has for him or he has for her. Even if there is an event of unfaithfulness, this love, though strained or broken, will persist. This is the nature of agape in a marital relationship, made possible only because God has endowed us with the gift of love.

The parent-child relationship is another which has or should have agape quality. No matter what poor choices offsprings make in life, they should still be the recipients of unbroken agape—strained, yes, but not broken or crushed to the point of nonexistence. In working with parents here and there in my professional career, I have known parents who disavowed their love relationship with their child or children, if indeed it ever existed. Agape in the parent-child relationship may be wounded, bruised, or crushed—but it should not be extinguished.

Drawing on the statements of agape for God and neighbors, the latter must not be overlooked or skimmed over. First, there is the need to define who "the neighbors" are. Neighbors are not just those on our residential block. They are included; but others at a distance, however far from us, are not to be excluded. This distance may be in terms of blocks or miles. No matter who they are or where they live, they are our neighbors. This includes unidentified or identified persons in North Korea and Iran as well as persons in Kenya and Iceland. This includes persons in our immediate communities who have ethnic or linguistic differences. As the children sing, "red, yellow, black, and white..."—all persons made in God's image are to be loved. Of course this does not mean that we are to love the life-style or choices of leadership in North Korea or even those terrorists in Syria and Iraq; it does mean, however, that our neighbors are God-created persons who live anywhere and everywhere. They are to be recipients of God-endowed and God-directed love.

By the way, it is not to be overlooked, that the second of the two greatest commandments—love God and neighbors —adds an important qualifier: love yourself. In other words, self-love is not to rise above other-love; it is to be equal to other-love. Hard to achieve? Of course it is; but a goal to be honestly and sincerely worked toward as is the first command, "Love the Lord thy God with all thy heart, soul, and mind."

The premise of the aforementioned essays is that there are certain emotions which we have—guilt, fear, grief, anger, and anxiety—that we should not hold. But! Love is an emotion that we should have and never let go.

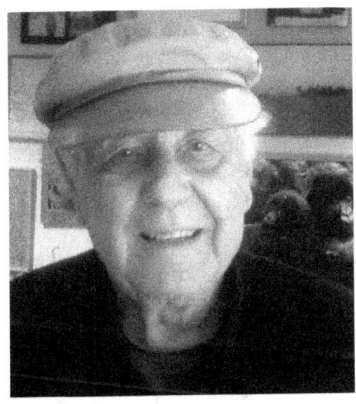

About the Author

Born to a humble family in Alvin, Texas during the Great Depression, Macklyn Ward Hubbell (known as Mickey) lost his father a few months before the attack on Pearl Harbor. His response to these hardships was to become an inquisitive extrovert who got a kick out of making people laugh. A popular athlete in high school, he dedicated his life to become a Christian minister at the age of sixteen. While attending Baylor University, he met Elizabeth Ann Melton (known as Bet), and they were married in 1951.

Though he embraced a spiritual path, Mickey also nurtured a deep respect for intellectual growth. After obtaining a B.A.

from Baylor, he went on to earn degrees from The University of Houston (M.A.), Southern Baptist Theological Seminary (B.D., Th.M.), and the University of Southern Mississippi (Ph.D.); so it came to pass that a bare-footed, fatherless boy who knew how it felt to wear burlap eventually became Dr. Macklyn Ward Hubbell, Professor Emeritus of New Orleans Baptist Theological Seminary.

Retired from his seminary position, Hubbell continues to minister as a pastor, counselor and civic leader. On the topic of mortality, he sums up his philosophy by saying, "I just want to **live** as long as I live—" approaching life with a youthful vigor and enthusiasm which inspires these traits in others.

In addition to loving his family, friends and neighbors across the globe, the author enjoys gardening, writing, and serving his local community in Cleveland, Mississippi. He has long enjoyed sharing his experiences and observations through his writing, and contributes a weekly column for The Bolivar Commercial, a local newspaper.

Published Works Include:

By Macklyn Ward Hubbell

Being a Good Senior Samaritan (1983)

Helping the Hurting (1988)

His daddy is God (1992)

On the Stoop (1993)

Who Me? Go Where? Do What? The Missionary and the Mission (1995)

Am I There Yet? (1999)

Outhouse Theology (2002)

This & That: A Collection of Mini-Essays (2004)

Frances from Louise (2004)

Goldman's Gold (2010)

Break Thou the Bread of Life (2013)

Above and Beyond Chance (2014)

Becoming One Flesh: A Marriage Primer (2014)

I Am There (2015)

Essays on Emotions: To Have and Not to Hold & To Have and to Hold (2016)

By Macklyn W. and Elizabeth M. Hubbell

Food in the Faubourgs: Dining in the Neighborhoods of New Orleans (1992)

Eating Up & Down the Delta (2006)

Artists Up & Down the Delta (2007)

Musicians Up and Down the Delta (2008)

Solomons Up & Down the Delta (2009)

U.S. Highway 61: A Travelogue: Up, Down, In Between, and In-Between In Between (2014)

By Elizabeth Melton Hubbell

Our Year at Ruschlikon, 1953-54: Letters from the Alps to the Delta (2016)

READER'S NOTES....

READER'S NOTES....